PANCREATITIS DIET PLAN GUIDE BOOK

The Complete Pancreatitis Diet Plan for Wellness: Dietary Approaches for Relief from Pancreatitis

REX LEWIS

Table of Contents

Introduction

A pancreatitis diet aims to facilitate the recovery of the pancreas and control symptoms related to pancreatitis, which is the inflammation of the pancreas. The pancreas is a gland that synthesizes digestive enzymes and insulin. Inflammation of the pancreas can result in a range of digestive problems and discomfort.

Below Are Some Overarching Principles For A Pancreatitis Diet:

1. A low-fat diet is strongly advised for those with pancreatitis. This aids in diminishing the stimulation of the pancreas, as the process of breaking

down fat necessitates the use of pancreatic enzymes. Refrain from consuming high-fat foods, including fried dishes, fatty meats, and full-fat dairy items.

Consuming smaller meals at regular intervals instead of three large meals can alleviate the burden on the pancreas and decrease the secretion of digestive enzymes.

3. Opt for lean sources of protein, such as skinless fowl, fish, and tofu. Restrict or abstain from consuming high-fat portions of meat and processed meat products.

4. Restrict Consumption of Refined Sugars and Sweets: Although it is

crucial to control blood sugar levels, consuming excessive amounts of refined sugars and sweets might worsen inflammation. Choose complex carbs derived from whole grains, fruits, and vegetables.

5. Maintaining proper hydration is essential, particularly when experiencing episodes of pancreatitis. It aids in the process of breaking down food and can assist to avoid issues such as excessive loss of body fluids.

6. Refrain from consuming alcohol: Alcohol has the potential to exacerbate pancreatitis, therefore it is crucial to completely eliminate or significantly restrict alcohol intake.

7. Restrict Caffeine Intake: Certain persons with pancreatitis may discover that caffeine worsens their symptoms. Monitor your level of tolerance and contemplate decreasing or completely stopping the consumption of caffeinated beverages.

8. Vitamins and Supplements: Occasionally, a healthcare physician may suggest particular vitamins or supplements to treat nutritional insufficiencies. Nevertheless, it is imperative that this be carried out under the guidance and oversight of a medical professional.

It is important to get guidance from a healthcare practitioner or a trained dietitian who can provide specialized counsel tailored to your specific condition. This is because the severity and causes of pancreatitis can differ across individuals. Furthermore, it is imperative to consult your healthcare team when making dietary modifications to ensure that your nutritional requirements are adequately addressed while effectively controlling pancreatitis.

CHAPTER ONE
What is Pancreatitis?

Pancreatitis is the inflammation of the pancreas, which is a gland located behind the stomach in the upper abdomen. The pancreas plays a crucial role in digestion and blood sugar regulation. It produces enzymes that help break down food in the small intestine and releases hormones, including insulin, to regulate blood sugar levels.

When the pancreas becomes inflamed, it can lead to various symptoms and complications. There are two main types of pancreatitis:

1. Acute Pancreatitis:

• Acute pancreatitis is a sudden and severe inflammation of the pancreas. It often occurs as a result of gallstones blocking the pancreatic duct or excessive alcohol consumption. Other causes can include certain medications, infections, trauma, or high levels of triglycerides (a type of fat) in the blood.

• Symptoms of acute pancreatitis may include severe abdominal pain, nausea, vomiting, fever, and an increased heart rate. Hospitalization may be required for treatment and monitoring.

2. Chronic Pancreatitis:

• Chronic pancreatitis is a long-term inflammation of the pancreas that can lead to permanent damage. It is often associated with prolonged alcohol abuse, but other causes may include genetic factors, certain medical conditions, or repeated episodes of acute pancreatitis.

• Symptoms of chronic pancreatitis can include persistent abdominal pain, weight loss, diarrhea, and malabsorption of nutrients. Treatment may involve managing symptoms, addressing nutritional deficiencies, and making lifestyle changes.

Common Risk Factors for Pancreatitis Include:

- **Gallstones:** These can block the pancreatic duct, leading to inflammation.

- **Alcohol Consumption:** Excessive alcohol intake is a significant risk factor for both acute and chronic pancreatitis.

- **Smoking:** Cigarette smoking increases the risk of pancreatitis.

- **Family History:** Genetic factors can contribute to an increased risk.

- **Certain Medical Conditions:** Conditions such as cystic fibrosis, hypertriglyceridemia, and autoimmune disorders can be associated with pancreatitis.

Diagnosis of pancreatitis often involves a combination of medical history, physical examination, blood tests, and imaging studies, such as CT scans or MRIs.

Treatment depends on the type and severity of pancreatitis but may include:

- **Pain Management:** Medications to alleviate pain.
- **Nutritional Support:** Dietary changes and, in some cases, nutritional supplements.
- **Management of Underlying Causes:** Addressing factors like alcohol consumption or gallstones.

- **Hospitalization:** In severe cases of acute pancreatitis, hospitalization may be necessary for supportive care.

It's essential for individuals experiencing symptoms or at risk for pancreatitis to seek medical attention promptly for proper diagnosis and management.

Types and Causes of Pancreatitis

Pancreatitis can be classified into two main types: acute pancreatitis and chronic pancreatitis. The causes of pancreatitis vary depending on the type, and both can have different contributing factors. Here's an overview of each type and their common causes:

1. Acute Pancreatitis:

Causes:

- **Gallstones:** One of the most common causes. Gallstones can block the pancreatic duct, leading to inflammation.
- **Alcohol Consumption:** Excessive alcohol intake can cause acute pancreatitis.
- **Trauma or Injury:** Physical trauma to the abdomen can trigger inflammation of the pancreas.
- **Infections:** Viral or bacterial infections, such as mumps or

certain parasites, can contribute.

- **Medications:** Certain medications, such as some antibiotics, steroids, and diuretics, may be associated with acute pancreatitis.

- **High Triglyceride Levels:** Elevated levels of triglycerides (a type of fat) in the blood can lead to pancreatitis.

- **Autoimmune Reactions:** In rare cases, the immune system may attack the pancreas.

2. Chronic Pancreatitis:

Causes:

- **Long-Term Alcohol Abuse:** A significant cause of chronic pancreatitis.

- **Smoking:** Cigarette smoking increases the risk of developing chronic pancreatitis.

- **Genetic Factors:** Inherited conditions, such as hereditary pancreatitis or cystic fibrosis, can contribute.

- **Recurrent Acute Pancreatitis:** Having multiple episodes of acute pancreatitis may lead to chronic inflammation.

- **Duct Blockages:** Conditions that cause blockages in the pancreatic duct, such as tumors or cysts.

- **Autoimmune Disorders:** Conditions where the immune system mistakenly attacks the pancreas.

It's important to note that in some cases, the exact cause of pancreatitis may not be identified (idiopathic pancreatitis).

Risk Factors for Pancreatitis:

- **Family History:** A family history of pancreatitis or certain genetic conditions.
- **Age:** Acute pancreatitis is more common in middle-aged and older adults, while chronic pancreatitis may develop over time.

- **Gender:** Men have a slightly higher risk of developing pancreatitis.

- **Certain Medical Conditions:** Conditions like hypertriglyceridemia, hypercalcemia, and autoimmune disorders may increase the risk.

Early diagnosis and appropriate management are crucial for both acute and chronic pancreatitis. Individuals experiencing symptoms such as severe abdominal pain, nausea, vomiting, and fever should seek medical attention promptly. Additionally, addressing underlying causes and making lifestyle changes can be essential in the prevention and management of pancreatitis. If you suspect pancreatitis, consult with a healthcare professional for a thorough evaluation and guidance.

Symptoms and Diagnosis

The symptoms of pancreatitis can vary depending on the type and severity of the condition. Here are the common symptoms associated with both acute and chronic pancreatitis:

Symptoms of Acute Pancreatitis:

- **Severe Abdominal Pain:** Sudden onset of intense, persistent pain in the upper abdomen that may radiate to the back.

- **Nausea and Vomiting:** Nausea and vomiting may accompany the abdominal pain.

- **Fever and Rapid Pulse:** Fever, increased heart rate, and other signs of systemic inflammation.

- **Tenderness or Swelling of the Abdomen:** The abdomen may feel tender or swollen to the touch.

- **Loss of Appetite:** Decreased appetite or aversion to eating.

- **Jaundice (in some cases):** Yellowing of the skin and eyes may occur if the pancreatitis is severe and involves blockage of the bile duct.

Symptoms of Chronic Pancreatitis:

• **Persistent Abdominal Pain:** Recurrent or persistent dull pain in the upper abdomen that may radiate to the back.

• **Weight Loss:** Unintentional weight loss due to malabsorption of nutrients.

• **Diarrhea or Greasy Stools:** Frequent diarrhea or stools that are greasy, bulky, and foul-smelling.

• **Nausea and Vomiting:** Nausea and vomiting may occur, particularly after eating fatty foods.

• **Malnutrition:** Deficiencies in essential nutrients due to impaired digestion and absorption.

• **Diabetes (in some cases):** Chronic pancreatitis can lead to damage to the insulin-producing cells in the pancreas, resulting in diabetes.

Diagnosis:

• **Medical History and Physical Examination:** A healthcare provider will ask about your symptoms, medical history, and any risk factors for pancreatitis. They will also perform a physical examination to assess for signs of abdominal tenderness or swelling.

• **Blood Tests:** Blood tests may be conducted to assess levels of pancreatic enzymes such as amylase and lipase, which are typically elevated in pancreatitis. Other blood tests may evaluate liver function and assess for signs of inflammation.

• **Imaging Studies:** Imaging tests such as ultrasound, computed tomography (CT) scan, or magnetic resonance imaging (MRI) may be used to visualize the pancreas and detect signs of inflammation, blockages, or other abnormalities.

• **Endoscopic Procedures:** In some cases, endoscopic retrograde cholangiopancreatography (ERCP) or endoscopic ultrasound (EUS) may be performed to evaluate the pancreatic ducts and obtain tissue samples for biopsy.

• **Other Tests:** Additional tests may be conducted to rule out other potential causes of abdominal pain or to assess for complications of pancreatitis.

Early diagnosis and prompt treatment are crucial for managing pancreatitis effectively and preventing complications. If you experience symptoms suggestive of pancreatitis, it's important to seek medical attention for a thorough evaluation and appropriate management.

CHAPTER TWO
The Significance of Diet in Pancreatitis

Nutrition is essential in the treatment of pancreatitis. Regardless of whether it is acute or chronic pancreatitis, following the appropriate nutritional plan is crucial for relieving symptoms, promoting the healing process, and avoiding complications. The significance of nutrition in pancreatitis can be attributed to several fundamental factors:

1. Alleviating Pancreatic Strain: Adhering to a low-fat diet reduces the activation of the pancreas. Restricting dietary fat lessens the burden on the pancreas since it generates digestive enzymes, specifically lipase, which is essential for fat breakdown. Preventing further inflammation is especially crucial in cases of both acute and chronic pancreatitis.

2. Symptom Management: Implementing a meticulously designed dietary regimen can effectively alleviate symptoms such as abdominal pain, nausea, and vomiting. For instance, refraining from consuming specific trigger foods and choosing readily digestible alternatives can help alleviate symptoms.

3. Preventing Malnutrition: Pancreatitis can result in impaired absorption of nutrients, hence contributing to the development of malnutrition. An intricately planned diet guarantees that the individual get sufficient nourishment, vitamins, and minerals. It is vital to prevent weight loss, deficits, and promote general health.

4. Chronic pancreatitis can result in impaired insulin production, which can lead to diabetes and disrupt blood sugar regulation. Regulating carbohydrate consumption and opting for complex carbs aids in maintaining stable blood sugar levels.

5. Abstaining from alcohol and caffeine is crucial for persons with pancreatitis, especially those with a previous history of alcohol-related pancreatitis. Moreover, certain individuals may discover that caffeine worsens symptoms, and reducing its consumption can be advantageous.

6. To prevent complications related to pancreatitis, specific dietary decisions might be made. Restricting the consumption of fat decreases the likelihood of producing gallstones, which can lead to the occurrence of pancreatitis.

7. Facilitating Healing: A diet abundant in essential nutrients enhances the process of healing. Sufficient amounts of protein, vitamins, and minerals are necessary for the process of tissue repair and the maintenance of overall health.

8. Weight Management: It is crucial for individuals with chronic pancreatitis to maintain an optimal weight. Maintaining a well-balanced diet is crucial for attaining and maintaining a healthy body weight, hence reducing issues associated with both being underweight and overweight.

9. Personalized Methodology: The effect of nutrition can differ among persons. Hence, it is imperative to collaborate with a healthcare expert or a qualified dietitian in order to develop a personalized nutritional regimen. This strategy takes into account the seriousness of the ailment, dietary requirements, and any particular triggers or sensitivities.

It is crucial to acknowledge that dietary guidelines may differ depending on the particular kind and severity of pancreatitis. It is important to seek guidance from healthcare experts, such as a gastroenterologist or a certified dietitian, in order to obtain individualized counsel that is specific to your particular situation. It is advisable to make dietary adjustments under their supervision to ensure that nutritional requirements are fulfilled while effectively controlling pancreatitis.

Dietary Guidelines for Pancreatitis

The Dietary Guidelines For Pancreatitis Aim To Alleviate Pancreatic Stress, Effectively Manage Symptoms, And Promote Overall Well-Being.

Below Are Some Overarching Dietary Guidelines For Patients With Pancreatitis:

1. Low-Fat Diet:

- Emphasize a low-fat diet to reduce the workload on the pancreas. Limit intake of fried foods, fatty meats, full-fat dairy products, and high-fat snacks.

2. Lean Proteins:

- Choose lean protein sources such as skinless poultry, fish, tofu, and legumes. Limit or avoid red meat and processed meats.

3. Small, Frequent Meals:

- Opt for smaller, more frequent meals throughout the day instead of three large meals. This helps prevent overstimulation of the pancreas.

4. **Hydration:**

- Stay well-hydrated by drinking plenty of water. Adequate hydration supports digestion and helps prevent complications like dehydration.

5. **Limit Refined Sugars and Sweets:**

- While managing blood sugar levels is important, excessive intake of refined sugars and sweets can exacerbate inflammation. Choose complex carbohydrates from whole grains, fruits, and vegetables.

6. Avoid Alcohol:

- Completely abstain from alcohol, especially if alcohol-related pancreatitis is a concern.

7. Limit Caffeine:

- Monitor your tolerance to caffeine. Some individuals may find that caffeine worsens their symptoms, and reducing or eliminating caffeinated beverages may be beneficial.

8. Vitamins and Minerals:

- Ensure adequate intake of vitamins and minerals, especially if there are deficiencies. This may involve incorporating a variety of fruits and vegetables into the diet or taking supplements under medical supervision.

9. Individualized Approach:

- Work with a healthcare professional or a registered dietitian to create an individualized dietary plan based on your specific condition, nutritional needs, and lifestyle.

10. Nutritional Supplements (If Needed):

- In some cases, individuals with pancreatitis may require nutritional supplements, especially if malabsorption is a concern. This should be done under medical supervision.

11. Monitor Triggers:

- Pay attention to specific foods that may trigger symptoms and consider eliminating or limiting them from your diet.

12. **Gradual Introduction of Foods:**

- After an episode of acute pancreatitis, it's often recommended to introduce solid foods gradually, starting with easily digestible options.

It's important to note that these guidelines provide a general overview, and individual needs may vary. Always consult with healthcare professionals, such as a gastroenterologist or a registered dietitian, to receive personalized advice based on your specific condition and circumstances. Regular monitoring and adjustments to the diet may be necessary as the condition evolves.

CHAPTER THREE
Building a Balanced Diet

Constructing a well-rounded diet entails including a diverse range of food that is high in nutrients, in the right amounts, to fulfill your body's requirements for energy, vitamins, minerals, and other vital nutrients. Below are fundamental principles for establishing a well-balanced diet:

1. Incorporate A Diverse Range Of Food Groups:

• **Produce:** Strive for a diverse assortment of colors to guarantee a wide array of vitamins and antioxidants.

• Opt for whole grains such as brown rice, quinoa, whole wheat, oats, and whole-grain bread to obtain dietary fiber and long-lasting energy.

• Protein sources should consist of lean meats, poultry, fish, eggs, legumes, nuts, and seeds. Ensure a comprehensive amino acid profile by diversifying protein sources.

• **Dairy or Dairy Alternatives:** Incorporate calcium and vitamin D-rich products, such as milk, yogurt, and fortified plant-based substitutes.

2. Control Portion Sizes:

• Exercise caution when it comes to portion sizes in order to prevent excessive consumption. Utilize smaller plates and pay attention to the hunger and fullness signals from your body.

3. Select lean protein sources in order to minimize the consumption of saturated fat. Incorporate fish, skinless poultry, legumes such as beans and lentils, and tofu into your diet.

4. Integrate Nutritious Fats:

• Include nutritious sources of fats, such as avocados, nuts, seeds, olive oil, and fatty seafood like salmon. Reduce the consumption of saturated and trans fats commonly found in fried foods and processed snacks.

5. Reduce the consumption of meals and drinks that contain significant amounts of added sugars. Exercise caution while consuming salt and choose whole, minimally processed meals instead.

6. Maintain Proper Hydration:

• Consume ample amounts of water throughout the day. Restrict the use of beverages high in sugar and excessive amounts of caffeine.

7. Take into Account Nutrient Timing:

• Distribute your meals and snacks evenly throughout the day to sustain a steady level of energy. Ensure that each meal has a balanced combination of macronutrients, including carbohydrates, proteins, and fats.

8. Foods with High Fiber Content:

• Ensure an ample intake of fiber through the consumption of fruits, vegetables, whole grains, and legumes in order to promote digestion and sustain a healthy gastrointestinal system.

9. Practice mindful eating by consciously attending to your sensations of hunger and fullness. Consume your food at a leisurely pace, relishing every mouthful, and refrain from being distracted by devices such as televisions or smartphones when eating.

10. Moderation and Balance:

• Consume a diverse range of meals in appropriate quantities. Striking a balance is crucial for fulfilling your dietary requirements without over consuming any specific vitamin.

11. Customize to Individual Requirements:

• Tailor your dietary choices according to your unique requirements, daily routine, and any particular medical issues. It is advisable to seek guidance from a certified dietician for individualized recommendations.

12. Regular Physical Activity:

• To achieve optimal health and well-being, it is important to engage in regular physical activity in addition to maintaining a balanced diet.

It is important to keep in mind that each person's dietary requirements can differ depending on factors such as age, gender, amount of physical activity, and any existing health concerns. It is recommended to get advice from a healthcare practitioner or a certified dietitian for specialized information that is tailored to your specific circumstances.

Pancreatitis-Friendly Recipes

When developing recipes suitable for individuals with pancreatitis, it is crucial to prioritize low-fat alternatives, ingredients that are readily digestible, and meals that are soft on the pancreas.

Below are some recipe suggestions that are appropriate for folks with pancreatitis:

1. Baked Salmon with Quinoa and Steamed Vegetables:

Ingredients:

- Salmon fillets
- Quinoa

- Mixed vegetables (zucchini, carrots, bell peppers)
- Olive oil
- Lemon juice
- Herbs and spices (such as dill or parsley)

Instructions:

1. Season salmon fillets with herbs, spices, and a drizzle of olive oil.
2. Bake salmon in the oven until cooked.
3. Cook quinoa according to package instructions.
4. Steam mixed vegetables.
5. Serve salmon over a bed of quinoa and steamed vegetables, drizzle with lemon juice.

2. **Chicken and Vegetable Stir-Fry:**

Ingredients:

- Chicken breast, thinly sliced
- Mixed stir-fry vegetables (broccoli, bell peppers, snap peas)
- Low-sodium soy sauce
- Ginger and garlic (minced)
- Brown rice or quinoa

Instructions:

1. Sauté chicken in a non-stick pan with ginger and garlic until cooked.
2. Add mixed vegetables and stir-fry until crisp-tender.
3. Season with low-sodium soy sauce.

4. Serve over cooked brown rice or quinoa.

3. **Vegetable and Lentil Soup:**

Ingredients:

- Mixed vegetables (carrots, celery, potatoes)
- Red lentils
- Low-sodium vegetable broth
- Herbs and spices (such as thyme and bay leaves)

Instructions:

1. Sauté vegetables in a pot until softened.
2. Add red lentils and vegetable broth.
3. Simmer until lentils are cooked.

4. Season with herbs and spices.

5. Serve as a nourishing soup.

4. Oatmeal with Banana and Almond Butter:

Ingredients:

- Old-fashioned oats
- Water or low-fat milk
- Ripe banana, sliced
- Almond butter

Instructions:

1. Cook oats with water or low-fat milk according to package instructions.

2. Top with sliced banana and a dollop of almond butter.

5. **Greek Yogurt Parfait:**

Ingredients:

- Greek yogurt (low-fat)
- Fresh berries (blueberries, strawberries)
- Granola (low-fat and low-sugar)

Instructions:

1. Layer Greek yogurt with fresh berries.
2. Top with a sprinkle of low-fat, low-sugar granola.

6. **Mashed Sweet Potatoes with Turkey:**

Ingredients:

- Sweet potatoes, peeled and cubed
- Ground turkey
- Olive oil
- Herbs and spices (such as rosemary and thyme)

Instructions:

1. Boil or steam sweet potatoes until soft.
2. Mash with a drizzle of olive oil.
3. Sauté ground turkey with herbs and spices until cooked.
4. Serve mashed sweet potatoes topped with seasoned turkey.

Always tailor recipes to individual preferences and dietary tolerances. It's advisable to consult with a healthcare professional or a registered dietitian for personalized advice based on the specific needs and tolerances of individuals with pancreatitis.

CHAPTER FOUR
Importance of Hydration

Adequate hydration is essential for maintaining optimal health and well-being, and it plays a significant role in several aspects associated to pancreatitis. The need of water cannot be overstated, particularly for patients suffering from pancreatitis.

1. Enhances Digestive Function:

• Sufficient hydration facilitates optimal digestive function, including the production of pancreatic enzymes essential for food processing. It guarantees that these enzymes exist in adequate amounts to efficiently decompose nutrients.

2. Mitigates Dehydration:

• Pancreatitis, especially during acute bouts, can result in fluid depletion through emesis, diarrhea, or reduced fluid consumption due to symptoms such as stomach discomfort and nausea. Ensuring adequate water is crucial in order to avoid dehydration, which can worsen symptoms and result in consequences.

3. Facilitates Healing:

• Adequate hydration enhances the body's inherent healing mechanisms, such as tissue restoration and rejuvenation. It guarantees that cells have the essential nutrients and oxygen required for optimal functioning, so aiding in the recuperation from inflammation and damage caused by pancreatitis.

4. Mitigates the Risk of Complications:

• Dehydration can heighten the likelihood of complications linked to pancreatitis, such as disturbances in electrolyte levels, renal issues, and hypovolemic shock. Ensuring sufficient water levels helps reduce these hazards and promotes general well-being.

5. Relieves Symptoms:

• Maintaining proper hydration will help relieve symptoms frequently linked to pancreatitis, such as abdominal pain, bloating, and discomfort. Additionally, it can perhaps mitigate the intensity of nausea and vomiting.

6. Promotes Kidney Function:

• Adequate hydration is crucial for optimal kidney function and aids in the prevention of issues such as kidney stones and urinary tract infections. These complications might arise as a result of pancreatitis or dehydration.

7. Improves Nutrient Assimilation:

• Adequate hydration facilitates the efficient assimilation of vital vitamins, minerals, and other nutrients from both food and supplements.

Malabsorption can occur in persons with pancreatitis, making it more crucial to address this issue.

8. Ensures Electrolyte Equilibrium:

• Sufficient hydration ensures the equilibrium of electrolytes in the body, which is essential for multiple physiological processes, including as neuron and muscle function, hydration level, and acid-base balance.

9. Promotes General Health and Well-being:

• Hydration is crucial for maintaining overall health and well-being, as it affects numerous bodily functions and systems. It aids in the regulation of body temperature, facilitates joint lubrication, enhances cardiovascular health, and fosters cognitive function.

10.   Personalized   Hydration Requirements:

• Hydration requirements can differ depending on variables such as age, sex, physique, level of physical activity, environmental conditions, and state of health. It is crucial to pay attention to the signals of thirst that your body sends and drink fluids consistently throughout the day.

Proper hydration is crucial for those with pancreatitis as it is essential for supporting digestive function, preventing dehydration, promoting healing, reducing the likelihood of complications, alleviating symptoms, and maintaining overall health and well-being. It is crucial to consume a sufficient quantity of liquids on a regular basis and be mindful of hydration requirements, particularly during instances of pancreatitis or exacerbations.

Tips for Dining Out with Pancreatitis

Managing symptoms successfully, it is feasible to enjoy meals outside the home while dealing with the challenges of dining out with pancreatitis through cautious choices and thinking. Below are some recommendations for those with pancreatitis when eating at a restaurant:

1. Conduct Preemptive Menu Research:

• Prior to visiting a restaurant, examine their menu online to locate choices that are compatible with a diet suitable for individuals with pancreatitis. Seek out foods that have a low fat content, are rich in lean protein, and contain readily digestible ingredients.

2. Convey your dietary requirements:

• Notify the restaurant personnel about your dietary limitations and pancreatitis condition. Inquire about the possibility of catering to your dietary requirements by creating meals with limited use of oil or butter and excluding fried or high-fat items.

3. Select Grilled or Baked Proteins:

• Opt for lean protein options that are cooked by grilling or baking rather than frying. Choices such as grilled chicken, fish, or tofu are frequently favorable options.

4. Request Modifications:

• Feel free to request modifications to dishes. Opt for steamed vegetables or a basic baked potato as a side dish instead of choosing fried choices. The majority of eateries are willing to cater to specific dietary needs.

5.   Select   Uncomplicated Preparations:

- Choose recipes that are straightforward, with a limited number of components and minimal use of seasonings. This decreases the probability of swallowing concealed fats or components that can elicit symptoms.

6. Refrain from consuming dishes that have creamy sauces, gravies, or dressings. These foods frequently contain a significant amount of fat and can potentially worsen symptoms of pancreatitis.

7. Regulate Portion Sizes:

• Contemplate requesting smaller servings or dividing foods to prevent excessive consumption. This enables you to savor the flavors without exerting excessive strain on your digestive system.

8. Select Low-Fat Side Dishes:

• If the restaurant has side dishes, choose low-fat alternatives like steamed vegetables, plain rice, or a basic salad with vinaigrette dressing.

9. Avoid Alcohol:

• Alcohol use might potentially trigger pancreatitis, hence it is advisable to abstain from consuming alcoholic beverages. Choose water, herbal tea, or other beverages that do not include alcohol or caffeine.

10. Include Enzyme Supplements in Your Packing List:

• If your healthcare physician suggests digestive enzyme supplements, take them before or during your meal to assist with digestion.

11. Exercise Caution with Spices:

• Certain spices and seasonings can potentially cause irritation to the digestive tract. If you have a sensitivity to specific spices, inquire about the seasoning utilized in a specific meal.

12. Be attuned to your body:

• Observe how your body reacts to various foods. If you see certain stimuli or feelings that cause a reaction or unease, make a mental or written record for future use.

13. Select Non-Irritating Liquids:

• Choose liquids that are non-caffeinated and non-acidic, such as water or herbal tea, to prevent potential irritations.

14. Carry Snacks:

• If there are limited options available, it is advisable to carry a small snack to complement your meal.

15. Strategy for Achieving Success:

• Select dining establishments renowned for their nutritious and adaptable menu choices. Engaging in advance preparation can enhance the overall satisfaction of a meal occasion.

It is important to seek guidance from a healthcare physician or a qualified dietician who can provide specialized recommendations tailored to your specific condition. It is essential to maintain a balance between indulging in dining out and making decisions that align with your pancreatitis-friendly diet.

Summary of Dietary Supplements

Supplements are products designed to enhance the diet by supplying extra nutrients or substances that may be deficient or inadequate in a person's normal diet. Although it is typically recommended to get nutrients from a balanced diet, supplements might be advantageous for persons with certain dietary limitations, deficits, or health issues. Below is a summary of prevalent categories of dietary supplements:

1. Multivitamins:

• Multivitamins consist of a blend of vital vitamins and minerals. They are specifically engineered to address possible deficiencies in nutrition and guarantee a minimum consumption of certain essential nutrients.

2. Vitamin and Mineral Supplements:

• These supplements include targeted vitamins (such as vitamin C, vitamin D, vitamin B complex) or minerals (such as calcium, iron, zinc) that may be deficient in the diet.

3. Omega-3 fatty acids commonly derived from fish oil, flaxseed oil, or algae, are supplements that include vital fatty acids. These fatty acids offer advantages for heart health, brain function, and the reduction of inflammation.

4. Probiotics:

• Probiotics consist of living helpful bacteria that can enhance a harmonious equilibrium of gut microbiota. They can provide benefits for gastrointestinal well-being and bolster the immune system.

5. Fiber supplements, such as psyllium husk or inulin, can aid in maintaining digestive health and regulating bowel motions, particularly for those who do not consume enough dietary fiber.

6. Calcium and Vitamin D supplements are commonly prescribed to promote optimal bone health. Calcium is required for the formation of bone structure, whilst vitamin D facilitates its absorption.

7. Iron Supplements:

• Iron supplements are typically prescribed for persons diagnosed with iron-deficiency anemia. It is crucial for the synthesis of hemoglobin in erythrocytes.

8. Folic Acid:

• Folic acid, a synthetic derivative of folate, plays a vital role in the creation of DNA and the division of cells. It is particularly crucial during pregnancy and for the purpose of averting neural tube abnormalities.

9. Vitamin B12 is essential for the synthesis of red blood cells and proper neurological functioning. Animal products are a common source of this substance, and supplements may be advised for individuals with deficits or specific dietary limitations.

10. Vitamin C:

- Vitamin C is crucial for collagen synthesis, wound healing, and immune system functionality due to its antioxidant qualities.

11. Magnesium:

- Magnesium plays a crucial role in multiple physiological processes, such as muscle and neuron activity, energy generation, and maintaining healthy bones.

12. Adaptogens are plants or chemicals that are thought to aid the body in adapting to stress and enhancing overall well-being. Some examples of these plants are ashwagandha and rhodiola.

13. Joint Supplements:

• Glucosamine and chondroitin sulfate are commonly used to promote joint health, especially in persons suffering from osteoarthritis.

14. Herbal Supplements:

• Echinacea, ginseng, and turmeric are among the herbal supplements that people use for their possible health advantages. Nevertheless, the effectiveness and safety of these products can differ, and it is important to be cautious.

15. Key Factors to Consider:

• It is imperative to seek advice from a healthcare expert before to initiating any supplement routine, as excessive consumption of specific vitamins and minerals might result in negative consequences.

• The requirement for supplements might differ across individuals depending on characteristics such as age, gender, health state, and diet.

• A well-balanced diet is still the fundamental way to receive vital nutrients.

It is advisable to consult healthcare specialists or qualified dietitians to ascertain the suitability of supplements for your individual requirements and health objectives.

Conclusion

In summary, pancreatitis is a medical illness distinguished by the inflammation of the pancreas, which can manifest as either acute or chronic. Treating pancreatitis requires a holistic approach, which includes medical intervention, adjustments to one's lifestyle, and dietary alterations. A pancreatitis-specific diet aims to minimize strain on the pancreas, effectively control symptoms, and proactively avoid complications.

Individuals with pancreatitis must strictly follow dietary restrictions that encompass:

1. Low-Fat Diet: Restricting the consumption of fat in order to lessen the burden on the pancreas.

2. Opt for lean protein sources to promote general well-being.

3. Balanced Meals: Consuming smaller, more frequent meals to prevent excessive stimulation of the pancreas.

4. Maintaining proper hydration is essential for promoting digestion and preventing dehydration.

5. Avoiding Triggers: Identifying and refraining from consuming foods that have the potential to cause symptoms.

6. Ensuring sufficient consumption of vitamins and minerals, potentially through the use of supplements under medical supervision.

When dining out with pancreatitis, it is important to carefully select menu items, communicate with restaurant staff, and make any alterations to accommodate dietary requirements. In order to properly manage symptoms, it is crucial to engage in advance planning, thoroughly investigate menus, and make well-informed decisions when it comes to enjoying meals.

Ensuring proper hydration is essential for maintaining digestive function, overall well-being, and minimizing complications related to pancreatitis, in addition to dietary factors. Sufficient hydration facilitates the body's healing mechanisms, mitigates the likelihood of dehydration, and relieves symptoms.

Although supplements might provide advantages for individuals with particular nutritional requirements or deficits, it is crucial to approach supplementation with prudence and under the supervision of healthcare experts. Supplements should serve as a supplement to a well-balanced diet, rather than serving as a replacement for it.

To effectively manage pancreatitis, it is important to take a comprehensive strategy. This includes working closely with healthcare specialists, following dietary guidelines, making thoughtful decisions while eating out, and ensuring proper hydration. Individuals suffering with pancreatitis should see healthcare professionals or trained dietitians for specialized guidance in developing a customized plan that caters to their specific requirements and promotes their overall health.

THE END